Running

How to Start Running to Lose Weight, Get Fit and Relieve Stress

Linda H. Harris

The trademarks that are used are without any consent, and the publication of the trademark is without permission or backing by the trademark owner. All trademarks and brands within this book are for clarifying purposes only and are owned by the owners themselves, not affiliated with this document.

ISBN: 978-1-64842-116-7

Table of Contents

Chapter 1: Why We Run – Introduction of Running

This introduction of running is meant to show you why people run. According to statistics from Running USA, the number of people who call themselves runners has been growing and there's also a sharp increase of people willing to run road races. There are a number of reasons for why this is becoming so popular as an exercise.

First, it's good for you. Running increases your heart rate, it burns calories and it strengthens a number of key muscle groups in your legs, hips and core. You'll also maximize your calorie burn by running. Jogging at a comfortable pace will help you burn about eight calories a minute. People who run tend to live healthier lives in general. When you're running on a regular basis, you're probably less likely to spend hours in front of the television binging on junk food.

Another reason running makes sense is that you can do it anywhere. You can run outdoors in the sunshine or in the dark. You can run on a treadmill if you hate the rain or the heat. You can run when you're on vacation, taking a day off or visiting your mother. It can also be a social activity. Running with a partner will hold you accountable to doing it and you can even meet new people while you're out running through the park or banking miles at the gym. If you prefer to do it alone, that's cool too. Or, you can bring your dog along.

There are mental benefits to running as well. Many people run in order to clear their minds, release stress and remove themselves from situations that cause anxiety. The endorphins you release while running will improve your mood and give you a healthier, happier outlook on life. Studies have even shown that running can improve your chances of avoiding dementia. It helps with your memory and might even protect you against Alzheimer's.

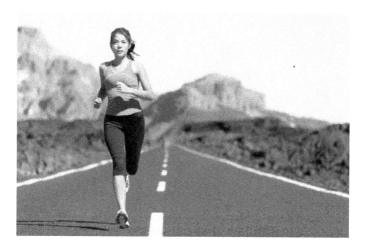

Self esteem is also known to skyrocket when you start calling yourself a runner. Even if you're only managing to get through a mile a day, getting that run completed gives you a lot of motivation to meet other goals. Your energy levels will increase as well, helping you to beat back that mid-afternoon slump that can strike while you're at work or trying to study.

Your body's bones will benefit from running. It's a high impact form of exercise, which means it will build the muscles you need to help you keep your bones stronger as you age. Finally, it will help you sleep better as well. Falling into bed exhausted and ready to shut down is a lot easier to do when you've spent a few hours picking up the pace and running.

This introduction of running should tell you that there are many good reasons to run. Whether you want to get healthier mentally, lose some weight or obtain a stronger physical body, running is a good way to reach those goals. You'll find yourself looking and feeling better and before too long, you'll be hooked on this exercise and recreational pastime. The rest of this book will show you how to start running, how to train for a race, and how to develop an eating plan that keeps pace with your running routine.

Chapter 2: Getting Started – Running Exercises and Techniques

The key to sticking with a successful running routine is to start small and build your way towards loftier goals. The strongest and most dedicated runners didn't start out by sprinting 10 miles every day. Start with a manageable pace and distance and then try to improve each week. These running exercises and techniques will help you get started and stay motivated.

Warming Up and Cooling Down

First, you need to know how to prepare your body for consistent running schedules. If this is your first time running or you haven't been physically active in a long time, your body will need to adapt to the work you're giving it. Warming up is a great way to get your muscles and your joints ready for the exercise and the physical demands. It protects you against injuries that can occur if you aren't careful and you're not aware of your body's capabilities and limitations.

The best warm ups for running will involve stretching your calves, rolling your ankles and doing a few squats and lunges to stretch out your leg muscles. Dynamic stretches, where you are moving while you stretch, are more beneficial than static stretches, where you'll stand still in the same position. You also want to walk for a few minutes before you begin running. This will get your heart ready for an increased rate and it will put your body through the motions; ensuring there isn't too much shock to your system when you really start to move.

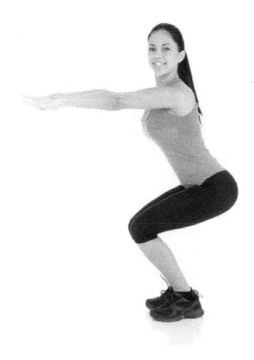

To cool down, you'll do many of the same things that you did while warming up. The purpose of a cool down after running is also to prevent injuries; stopping your muscles suddenly from moving and pushing can be damaging and could lead to cramping, sprains and strains. Once you've completed your run, walk for about two or three minutes to bring your heart rate down and regulate your breathing. Then, do a few lunges or squats to stretch out your legs and hips. Walk on the balls of your feet for 30 seconds to help your calves cool down.

Form and Technique: How to Run

The key to maximizing your speed as well as your distance when you run is your form. Running with the proper form can also protect you from injuries and give you a better physical and mental workout. If you run the wrong way, you're going to get into bad habits that are hard to break. Pay attention to your form, and use a few techniques while you're running to ensure that you're doing it properly.

Your running technique will depend on your size, strength and flexibility. What works for one runner won't necessarily work for every runner and you need to make sure you're focused on comfort and safety. If you remember these important techniques, you'll be sure to run correctly.

Pushing up and off the ground is the way you want to start and maintain a stride. Think of leaving the ground behind you as you run in order to ensure that your feet are doing what they need to do to keep the rest of your body moving.

Keep your stride short and fast. You don't want to do any leaping. You also don't want to think about distance right now. Take short, fast steps while you run in order to find the right pace and keep good form.

Put your foot right below your knee. The leg should be in a straight line, with the foot coming down onto the ground right underneath where your knee is located. If your foot is reaching out in front of where your knee is, you're setting yourself up for a potential injury. Don't worry about toe/heel or heel/toe. It doesn't matter which part of your foot hits the ground first, as long as it's lined up under your knee.

Bend your elbows. If you've ever seen anyone running with their arms straight down by their sides, you know it looks weird. It's also counterproductive to running for exercise. Bend your elbows and hold them at your sides at 90 degree angles.

Keep your head and your chest up, ensuring that you aren't bending over at the waist. Hold your shoulders back and keep your eyes focused on what's ahead of you. Let your hands relax. You don't want to ball them into fists or let them flail around while you run. They should just be loose and level with your midsection.

Training Plan: Two Weeks

Running well for two weeks will set you up on a path that keeps you motivated and goal-oriented. You aren't running any races or marathons yet, so use the first two weeks as a time to get comfortable with the act of running and to work on the running exercises and techniques that will help your form.

Week 1: Walking and Running

During the first week, you want to concentrate on how your body feels while it's running. Too much running will leave you feel discouraged and impatient, so you'll combine running and walking to build yourself up for the second week. Running every day might be difficult as a beginner, so set a goal of running four or five days in the first week. On the days that you don't run, take a long and brisk walk so that you keep yourself active and your body moving.

You will need something that can keep track of your time. This might be a stopwatch, a cell phone or even a fitness device that you can wear on your wrist or your clothing. Make sure you stay hydrated. It might be hard to carry water while you're running, but have some ready for when you're finished.

Start with a goal of 30 minutes. In the first week, you will split that time between running and walking. Start with five minutes of brisk, aerobic walking. Then, run for five minutes. You don't have to run fast. As long as you've picked up the pace to be something more than your walk, you're doing great. After five minutes, slow down to a walk, but keep your walking pace elevated so that you aren't at a complete stroll. After five minutes of walking, you'll do another five minutes of running. Slow down again to the walking and keep alternating between five walking minutes and five running minutes until you've completed a solid half hour of running.

Week Two: Increase the Running

If you found it really hard to keep up with the five minutes of walking and then five minutes of running, stick with that same schedule again for the second week. Keep at it until it seems more manageable for you. If the alternating five minutes of running and walking was a breeze or you feel like you can challenge yourself more, you're ready to move onto a pace that requires more running time and less walking time.

Start with the five minute walk, but this time you'll increase your running time to 10 minutes. Just like in the first week, you don't need to run hard or fast, you just need to run. After those 10 minutes, walk again for another five minutes and then finish out the half hour with another 10 minutes of running. Don't forget to cool down with some walking and some stretching.

As you move from week to week, you want to reduce the number of minutes you spend walking and increase the number of minutes you spend running. It's a simple plan that allows you to build your endurance, strength and ability. Before too long, you'll spend the entire 30 minutes in a run.

Where to Run: Outdoor Running and Treadmills

As you know, one of the benefits of running as exercise is that you can do it anywhere. It's also both an indoor and an outdoor sport.

Maybe you prefer to run outside on pavement, sand or through the park. Or, perhaps you're an indoor person with little tolerance for the heat and the rain and all the other elements, and you prefer to workout on a treadmill. Either option brings you just as much physical activity, so do what works best for you. There are a few things you need to know about running exercises and techniques in each location.

Outdoor running often provides a scenic backdrop that can help you forget that your lungs are burning and your legs are rubbery. Make sure you're aware of your terrain. When you run outside, you're not always running on even pavement. There are dips and holes and rocks and debris that can get in your way and trip you up. Pay attention to your surroundings so you know what dangers might be lurking. You will also need to be flexible with your stride. On a treadmill, you're able to fall into a consistent stride but when you run outside, you need to prepare for sharp turns, sudden hills and the resistance of wind. You'll need to tweak your stride while you're running, which means slowing down and speeding up and occasionally jumping out of the way.

Think about weather elements as well. Layers are great and material that protects you from rain and wind will also go a long way in keeping you comfortable. Don't forget your hat, sunglasses and sunscreen when you're running under the strong summer sun.

Treadmill running can be a bit more consistent. You're basically setting your pace and your terrain on the machine. Make sure you're getting enough exertion. It can be tempting to set the controls at a simple pace and then just cruise through your run without breaking a sweat. That's not what you want. Set a pace that will keep you challenged. You also have the benefit of using inclines. Create your own hills and program them in to arrive at different intervals so you get to use your leg muscles and core while you're running.

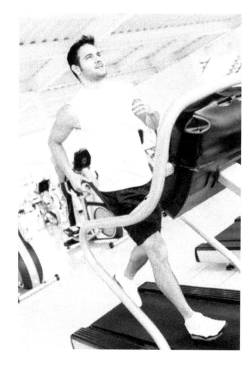

Treadmill running can be better at preventing injuries. You don't have to worry about weather issues or bumps in the road. The impact on the machine's belt is also easier on your joints than the force of real ground outside. If you're recovering from an injury or a total beginner, running on a treadmill can usually be much safer for you than running outside.

Mindful Running: Getting the Most from Your Exercise

Naturally, most people run for the physical benefits. There is a lot to be gained for your heart health, weight management and overall health when you adopt a consistent running routine. However, there are also a number of mental and emotional benefits to running. Not only can you beat back the potential for depression and stress, you can also use your running time to get in touch with your inner self and to increase your mindfulness. Being mindful while you run can help you sort out problems; using your subconscious to be present in the moment and focused on the really important things you have going on inside your mind and body.

Mindful running can happen naturally if you pay attention to a few key things. First, focus on your breathing. Inhale through your nose if you can, and allow your breathing to fall into the same pattern as your steps. The result will be meditative. Once your breathing is synced, look at your stride. Pay attention to how your feet look, sound and feel. Visualize yourself being pulled forward as you run, and let your mind get quiet while you find your balance and your inner peace. This is mindful running and you'll find even better stress reduction benefits when you exercise this way.

These running exercises and techniques should get you started in the right direction. Whether you're doing this because you want to exercise more, because you want to run in your first 5K or because you know it's good for your mind and body, running can have a great and positive impact on your life.

Chapter 3: How to Train for Your First Race

Running in a race is a good way for you to access the social benefits of running. While a race usually indicates that you're competing against a field of other runners, you're not really competing against them as much as you're competing with them. Your goal should not really be to win the race (although that would be wonderful). Your goal is to improve your own personal best. Steadily improving your recorded running time is a great reason to enter races. Many people enjoy running in races to feel like part of a team or even to raise money for charity. Whatever your reasons for running in a race, you need to prepare yourself. If you're wondering how to train for your first race, the answer is fairly simple: you practice.

Choosing a Race

First, you need to choose the right race. Take a look at the distance first. The most common type of road race is the 5K, and it works well for beginners as well as experienced runners. If you have been running for a long time and you're finally ready to start entering races, you might be okay in a 10K. That's your own decision, but make sure you're choosing a distance that you're likely to finish. The only way not to win a race is by not crossing the finish line.

In addition to looking at distance, you need to consider the race route. If there are a lot of hills and uneven terrain, you need to be prepared for it. You also need to be prepared for weather; running a 5K in Miami in August will be a lot different than running in New York in January. Your first race should be in a place that feels familiar to you. One of the best things about running races is that you get to go to new places. However, for your first race you want to feel comfortable with the climate, terrain and the general area that you'll be covering.

How to Train for Your First Race

Assuming you decide to run a 5K for starters, you'll need to work your way up to running at least that distance in one single outing. If your running progression has only led you to completing a mile or two, you're going to have to increase what you run on a daily basis. The 5K race you enter will equal just over three miles. If you're not sure you can run three miles every day - that's okay. It doesn't mean you can't run in a 5K race. You don't have to run that distance every day, you simply have to run it one day - on the race day. However, you want to enter the race with the confidence that you can complete it.

As you're training, run at least three miles one day per week. Even if you only run one mile three days a week, try to get that three mile run in on one day of the week. If you practice getting through the full three miles once a week, you'll know you can do it. Leading up to the race, follow your same training schedule. And if you do most of your running on a treadmill, get outside during the three mile run day so you'll be better prepared on race day.

Whether you run a 5K or a 10K or something in between, you'll enjoy the sense of accomplishment and community. Training simply means practicing, and if you practice your running on a consistent basis, you'll be ready. Track your time and try to improve with every race you win.

Chapter 4: Nutrition and Diet for Running

It's important to have an eating plan that keeps pace with your running routine. If you aren't eating the right nutrients and providing your body with the fuel that's necessary to keep you going, you'll have a hard time maintaining a consistent running schedule. If you're running in order to lose weight or become healthier, it's even more important to pay close attention to what you eat. Nutrition and diet for running requires a lot of protein to keep your muscles strong, complex carbohydrates that provide the energy you need to keep going, and of course all the fresh fruits and vegetables you can eat to keep your body in top physical form.

What to Eat: Best Foods for Runners

For runners, food is about more than taste and hunger. It's what brings energy to your body and you need to make strategic decisions when you're putting together a meal or a snack. Every calorie counts and you want to remember that instead of depriving your body, you want to fill it with everything good.

Peanut Butter is an excellent diet staple for runners. You get great protein and it's easy for your body to digest. It also tastes pretty good, especially when you eat it on toast or spread on apples and celery.

Bananas are also great. They are high in potassium, which is great for your blood pressure. It also protects you against cramping while you run. The carbohydrates that come with bananas are the good kinds of carbs - they provide energy instead of useless sugar.

Eat yogurt every day if you can. The running you do will help you strengthen your bones and the calcium in yogurt will assist with creating bone density, especially as you age. In addition to the calcium, you also get protein, which will help your muscles repair themselves between runs. Look for yogurt that is low in fat or fat free and don't eat anything with a lot of added sugars.

Protein is particularly important for runners. If you're a vegetarian, you'll want to make sure you get plenty of it from plant-based sources. Nuts are also excellent sources of protein and if you eat them - eggs and fish. If you're not a vegetarian, you'll want to add lean beef to your plate a few times a week. It's very high in protein and it also contains iron, which is necessary in runners to combat fatigue. If you have an iron deficiency, you'll find that your endurance and stamina will suffer. Salmon is another great protein source for runners. In addition to the protein there are omega-3 fatty acids, which will curb any inflammation you might get in your joints from running every day.

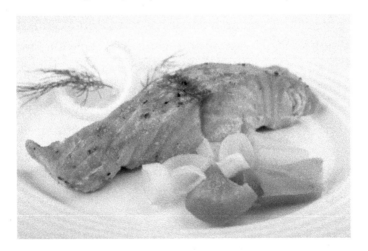

What to Eat: Before and After You Run

The food you eat before and after you run will make a big difference in how you feel while you're exercising and while you're recovering. It's not a good idea to eat a heavy meal right before a run, but you do want to make sure you'll have the energy you need to reach your goals.

About 30 minutes before you run, eat something that provides carbohydrates and protein. Peanut butter on a whole grain bagel is a great choice, or an English muffin with some almond butter and honey. Try some oatmeal if you run in the morning or have a small serving of pasta if you run later in the day. While eating foods high in fiber is generally good for runners, avoid high fiber foods and high fat foods before you go running. You want to stick with foods that are easy to digest.

After a run, it's all about recovery. You want to feed your body foods that will help repair muscles and soothe joints. Muscle soreness can set in if you aren't supplying your body with the necessary nutrients. Always restore your fluids as well. Drink a lot of water. Once you've replaced the fluids you've lost, fill up on protein. Have a grilled chicken breast with a salad or a heaping bowl of brown rice. Eat some scrambled eggs or an omelet with crisp seasonal veggies. If cooking something right after a run isn't possible, grab a container of yogurt, eat a banana and an apple or try some hummus with raw veggies like carrots and peppers.

What to Eat: Before a Race

Before a race, your stomach is probably fluttering with nerves, excitement and anticipation. You don't want to worry about running out of energy halfway through your 5K or half marathon. On the morning of your race, stick to the same foods you have been eating during your training runs. All the good proteins and carbohydrates like peanut butter, eggs and yogurt are great as fuel sources. A few days leading up to the race, concentrate on your protein intake and make sure you're getting enough. Chicken, beef, fish, eggs and pasta, rice and legumes are all good foods to get your body ready for race day. Stay away from anything processed or high in fats and sugars.

The nutrition and diet for running plan needs to focus on keeping your body strong. Even if you have begun running to lose weight, you don't want to be preoccupied with calories. Choose quality over quantity and put together an eating plan that complements your new fitness plans. Running puts you more in tune with your body - so you'll know what it needs.

Chapter 5: Running Tips for Beginners

These running tips for beginners are intended to keep you motivated and excited about your new fitness activity. Whether you're running to lose weight, to get stronger and healthier or because you want to enter a race, it's a great way to stay strong and active. Some of the most common mistakes that new runners make are easy to correct. These tips will help you avoid those mistakes altogether and keep you motivated, comfortable and safe. It's time to get excited about running!

What to Wear

There are some logistical considerations to sort out before you launch yourself into your running plans. The most important thing you need to know is probably what you should wear. This depends on your personal style and what makes you comfortable. It also needs to factor in where you're running and what kind of climate and terrain you're dealing with. When you run indoors or on a treadmill, you can wear anything you want, especially if you're in the privacy of your own home. But if you run outside, you'll need to plan for heat, cold, rain and wind. Dressing in layers is always a good idea. Choose fabrics that keep you dry and your body temperature regulated. In colder climates, don't forget gloves and jackets and hats and earmuffs. In hot weather, you'll want sunscreen and sunglasses and light clothing such as tank tops and shorts.

Footwear is very important. Buy shoes that are designed for running. You don't want a tennis shoe or a cross trainer. It has to handle the shock of running and protect your body from injuries. There should be a cushion in the heel and the toe area so your feet are protected against the impact of your body weight slamming down while you run. Running shoes will also help with traction and breathability.

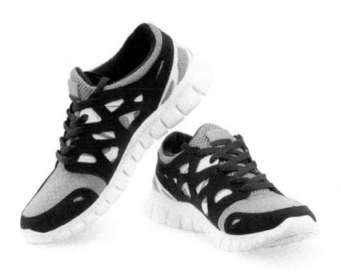

Try on a few different types of running shoes before you buy. Get an idea of what will feel best on your feet while you run. Feet come in many different shapes and sizes and the best running shoe for you will not necessarily be the best running shoe for your spouse or sibling. Your arch also dictates what you should put on your feet. If you have a high arch, you'll want something completely different than someone who is flat-footed. Try the shoes on and talk to the salespeople who are knowledgeable about running.

Developing a Plan

Serious runners like consistency. They like to develop a training plan and then they stick to their plan. Many runners build their entire day around their morning, afternoon or evening run. Take a look at your lifestyle and your day and figure out where a run will fit in. You want to give yourself plenty of time for warming up, running, cooling down and recovering. Decide what time of day you want to run and where you want to go. Once you have those things in place, you can begin to experiment with distance and location. Decide how far you want to run and how fast. Set goals, track your goals and stick to your program.

While having a consistent plan in place is very important, you also want to be flexible for when your life gets interesting. If you have to travel for work or vacation, make sure you can incorporate a run into those plans. Most hotels have fitness centers where you can run on a treadmill, or you can explore a new location and run out of doors.

Staying Motivated

Runners stay motivated in a number of ways. If you enjoy the social aspect of running, consider running with someone. This will help with motivation and keep you accountable to your running partner. There are even running clubs and leagues in many communities where you can run with a group of people. Write down your goals and track your progress. This is an excellent way to stay motivated because if you can see the progress you're making, you'll have the drive to keep improving. Consider entering a race, even if you think you're not ready yet. Knowing that you have a 5K coming up in a month or two will keep you on track and get you out the door and moving on a consistent basis.

Try mindful running. If you don't want to be too attached to the numbers involved in running - distance, time, etc., then you can simply use running as a way to find peace in an otherwise hectic day. Many people run in order to stay mentally balanced and to avoid depression, stress and anxiety. Running for sound emotional and mental health requires little motivation - you know it feels good, so you keep doing it. Be completely present in the moment while you run and don't worry about your time or your personal record or your upcoming race.

Avoiding Injuries

Nothing will throw you off your running course like an injury. It doesn't even have to be a big one - even a sprained ankle or a pulled muscle will leave you sore and unable to run for a week or two. Avoid injuries by wearing the right footwear, being mindful of your surroundings when you're outside running or on a treadmill and taking care of your body. Stay hydrated before, after and during your runs. Incorporate some strength training into your fitness plans. A stronger core will allow you to run with confidence. Warm up and cool down every time you run, even if you're just out for a slow jog. Finally, know your abilities and don't be afraid to respect your limitations. You don't have to run a marathon tomorrow. Take your time and build your skills.

These running tips for beginners should help you get started. You'll find running to be enjoyable, challenging and rewarding. Whether you're running for pleasure, health or competition, you're introducing a great habit into your life and it will impact you for years to come. Start small and keep moving towards greater goals.

Conclusion

Whether you want to lose some weight, obtain a stronger physical body or get healthier mentally, running is a great way to reach those goals. The key to sticking with a successful running routine is to start small and build your way towards loftier goals. I hope this book helps you start running, stay motivated and win your races.

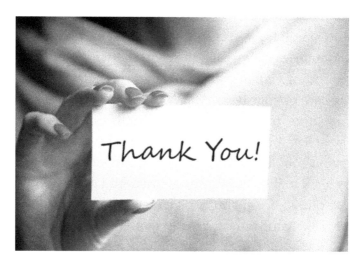

Finally, I want to thank you for reading my book. If you enjoyed the book, please share your thoughts and post a review on the book retailer's website. It would be greatly appreciated!

Best wishes,

Linda Harris

Check Out My Other Books

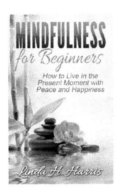

Mindfulness for Beginners: How to Live in the Present Moment with Peace and Happiness

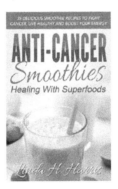

Anti-Cancer Smoothies: Healing With Superfoods
35 Delicious Smoothie Recipes to Fight Cancer, Live Healthy and Boost Your Energy

Lightning Source UK Ltd.
Milton Keynes UK
UKHW020634071220
374755UK00006B/668